TETRALOGY OF FALLOT

ALL THE PROCESSES OF HEALING

TETRALOGY OF THE FALLOT REVEALED

DR. CYRIL LAKES

Contents

CHAPTER ONE

INTRODUCTION

Tetralogy of Fallot is an uncommon ailment that arises from a confluence of four congenital cardiac abnormalities. Blood with low oxygen content flows from the heart and into the body as a result of several structural cardiac abnormalities. Tetralogy of Fallot patients typically have blue-tinged skin because not enough oxygen is circulating in their blood.

Tetralogy of Fallot is frequently identified in the early stages of life. However, depending on the severity of the problems and symptoms, tetralogy of Fallot may not be discovered until later in life. The majority of kids with tetralogy of Fallot lead quite normal lives provided they receive early diagnosis and adequate treatment; nonetheless, they may require ongoing medical attention and might not be able to move as much.

Symptoms

The degree of blood flow restriction from the right ventricle into the lungs determines the symptoms of telangiectomy. Among the symptoms and indicators are:

A blue tint to the skin brought on by low oxygen levels in the blood (cyanosis)

Breathing quickly and having trouble breathing, especially when eating

Unconsciousness (passing out)

Clubbing refers to the abnormally rounded form of the nail bed in fingers and toes.

Unsatisfactory weight growth

Easily fatigued while playing

Intolerance

Prolonged sobbing

A little murmur in the heart

Tet enchantments

Babies with tetralogy of Fallot occasionally wake up crying, eating, having a bowel movement, or kicking their legs, at which point their skin, nails, and lips become a deep blue color. These episodes, sometimes known as Tet spells, are brought on by a sharp decrease in blood oxygen levels. Younger children or toddlers may squat reflexively when they are out of breath. The lungs receive more blood when one is squatting. Tet episodes are more common in newborns between the ages of two and four months.

When to visit a physician

In the event that your child exhibits any of the following symptoms, get medical attention:

- breathing difficulties
- skin discolouration that is bluish
- fainting or having seizures
- Deficiency

- Unusual agitation

Should your infant turn blue (cyanotic), turn him or her onto the side and bring the knees up to the chest. By doing this, blood flow to the lungs is improved. Dial your local emergency number or 911 right away.

Reasons

Tetralogy of Fallot happens when the baby's heart is still forming during fetal growth. Tetralogy of Fallot is primarily caused by unknown sources, while risk factors like poor maternal nutrition, viral infection, or genetic diseases may enhance the condition's likelihood.

**The tetralogy of Fallot is composed of
the following four abnormalities:**

Stenosis of the pulmonary valve. The pulmonary valve, the flap that divides the heart's right ventricle from the pulmonary artery the major blood vessel that supplies the lungs is narrowing in this area. The pulmonary valve narrows, reducing the amount of blood that reaches the lungs. The muscle underlying the pulmonary valve may also be impacted by the constriction.

Septal defect in the ventricle. The two bottom chambers of the heart, known as the ventricles, are divided by this hole in the wall. The opening permits new oxygenated blood from the lungs to mix with deoxygenated blood from the right ventricle, which has traveled throughout the body and is on its way to the lungs to replace its oxygen supply. Inefficient blood flow occurs from the left ventricle back to the right ventricle. The body's supply of oxygenated blood is diluted by the blood's capacity to pass through the ventricular septal defect, which over time may damage the heart.

aorta in the lead. The main artery that leaves the body, the aorta, normally splits out from the left ventricle. When a person has tetralogy of Fallot, their aorta is positioned precisely above the ventricular septal defect and moved slightly to the right. The blood from the right and left ventricles enters the aorta in this position, combining the oxygen-rich blood from the left ventricle with the oxygen-poor blood from the right.

ventricular hypertrophy on the right. The heart's right ventricle's muscular wall thickens and enlarges when the pumping activity becomes strained. This may eventually lead to the heart stiffening, weakening, and failing.

Occasionally, infants with tetralogy of Fallot will also have an atrial septal defect, which is a hole between the upper chambers of the heart. The condition that results from this is called pentalogy of Fallot.

RISK ELEMENTS

Although the precise etiology of tetralogy of Fallot remains unclear, a number of variables may raise a baby's chance of being born with the disorder. Among them are:

- A maternal viral disease, such German measles, rubella, during pregnancy
- Alcoholism in mothers
- inadequate dietary intake
- a mother who is over 40
- A parent with Fallot tetralogy
- infants who also have DiGeorge syndrome or Down syndrome at birth

COMMITMENTS

Every infant diagnosed with tetralogy of Fallot requires corrective surgery. Your infant might not grow and develop normally if you don't treat them. Additionally, there is a higher chance of severe side effects, like infective endocarditis, which is an infection-related inflammation of the heart's inner lining.

If left untreated, tetralogy of Fallot cases typically lead to serious consequences over time, including the possibility of death or incapacity by early adulthood.

Getting Ready for Your Consultation

Most likely, you'll start by visiting a general practitioner or your family physician. That being said, a physician who specializes in heart issues (cardiologist) will be referred to you next.

Here are some tips to help you prepare for your visit and know what to anticipate from your physician.

What you're capable of

Read any restrictions about appointments in advance. Make careful to inquire about any necessary preparations, such as limiting your baby's diet, while scheduling the visit.

Note any symptoms your baby is exhibiting, even if they don't seem to be connected to the reason you made the appointment.

Record the baby's family history, incorporating as much information as possible from the father's and mother's sides.

CHAPTER TWO

If at all feasible, invite a friend or family member to accompany you. It might occasionally be challenging to recall everything that was said to you during an appointment. It can also be extremely distressing to hear that your child has a heart abnormality, which could make it more difficult for you to recall what the doctor says next. A companion of yours might pick up on details that you overlooked.

Make a list of questions for your child's physician

To maximize the time of your session, prepare a list of questions. Some fundamental inquiries to pose to your child's physician regarding tetralogy of Fallot include:

- What is my baby's most likely cause of symptoms?

- Exist any other plausible explanations for these symptoms?

- Which testing is my child in need of? Do you need to prepare in any way for these tests?

- Which of the available treatments would you suggest?

- What potential side effects are there from surgery?

- After surgery, what is the outlook for my child? Is he or she able to lead a typical life?

- There are additional medical issues with my child. How do I oversee them both the best I can?

- Does my child have to abide by any rules regarding what they can and cannot do?

- Can he or she participate in sports? Engage in gym activities?

- What caused this to occur?

- Will this occur in subsequent pregnancies as well?

- Is there a method to stop this from occurring?

- Are there any printed materials, such as brochures, available for me to take home?

- Which websites would you advise people to visit?

Do not be afraid to ask questions during your appointment if there is anything you don't understand, in addition to the questions you have planned to ask your doctor.

What to anticipate from your physician

- The doctor that examines your child will probably ask you a lot of questions, like:
- When did you initially observe the symptoms in your child?
- Do your child's symptoms come on all the time or only sometimes?
- Does your child's condition seem to be getting better?
- What seems to exacerbate your child's problems, if anything?

- How does your child sleep and eat?

- Have you observed episodes of fainting or a darker shade of blue or dusky complexion and lips on your child?

- Is your youngster losing weight or throwing up?

What you can accomplish in the interim

Here are some ideas to help your infant feel more comfortable as you wait for treatments and your doctor's appointment:

Give your infant a slow meal. Give him or her more frequent, smaller meals as well.

Throughout a Tet period, assist your child. Your child's lips, nails, and skin may become blue after they wake up, cry, or feed during a Tet episode. Your ability to maintain composure can assist your child feel less anxious. Gently lifting your child's knees to the chest will help increase blood flow to the heart and lungs.

Exams and diagnosis

If your newborn has blue-tinged skin or if there is a heart murmur in their chest (an irregular whooshing sound brought on by turbulent blood flow), the doctor may suggest tetralogy of Fallot. Your doctor can confirm the diagnosis with multiple testing.

chest radiography. An enlarged right ventricle is a common X-ray symptom of tetralogy of Fallot, giving the heart a "boot-shaped" appearance.

blood examination. A complete blood count, which counts every type of cell in the blood, is required for your child. When tetralogy of Fallot occurs, the body tries to raise the blood's oxygen content, which can lead to an excessively high red blood cell count (erythrocytosis).

Measurement of oxygen levels (pulse oximetry). This test measures the blood's oxygen content using a tiny sensor that is applied to a finger or toe.

echocardiography. Echocardiograms create an image of the heart by using high-pitched sound waves that are inaudible to human ears. Your baby's heart generates sound waves that can be seen on a video screen as moving pictures. This test aids in the diagnosis of tetralogy of Fallot by enabling the physician to determine the presence or absence of a ventricular septal defect, the normal construction of the pulmonary valve, the functionality of the right ventricle, and the correct positioning of the aorta.

ECG. Every time the heart contracts, the electrical activity in the heart is recorded by an ECG. Your kid will have patches containing wires, or electrodes, applied to their ankles, wrists, and chest during this surgery. Electrical activity is measured by the electrodes and recorded on paper. This test helps establish whether the heart rhythm is regular and whether your baby has ventricular hypertrophy, or an enlargement of the right ventricle.

catheterization of the heart. A tiny, flexible tube called a catheter is inserted by your doctor into your baby's groin vein or artery and threaded up to the heart during this surgery. To show the structures of your baby's heart on X-ray images, a dye is given through the catheter. In addition, the catheter gauges blood vessel and cardiac chamber pressure and oxygen saturation.

MEDICATIONS AND SUBTLES

The only proven treatment for tetralogy of Fallot is surgery. There are two kinds of surgery that can be done: an interim shunt treatment or an intracardiac repair. The majority of infants and kids will require intracardiac repair.

intracardiac replacement

The majority of infants with tetralogy of Fallot are treated with intracardiac repair, an open cardiac procedure. Usually, this procedure is done in the first year of life. In order to seal the opening between the ventricles, the surgeon covers the ventricular septal defect with a patch during this treatment. In order to improve blood flow to the lungs, he or she additionally expands the pulmonary arteries and fixes the restricted pulmonary valve. The blood's oxygen content rises during intracardiac repair, and your baby's symptoms will subside.

Interim surgery

Sometimes babies require an interim procedure in addition to intracardiac repair. Doctors will install a bypass (shunt) between the aorta and pulmonary artery if your child was born preterm or has hypoplastic, or undeveloped, pulmonary arteries. The lungs receive more blood flow thanks to this bypass. The shunt is taken out when your child is prepared for intracardiac repair.

Following the procedure

After intracardiac repair, the majority of newborns recover successfully, however problems might occur. Chronic pulmonary regurgitation, in which blood seeps through the pulmonary valve, and arrhythmia, or irregular heartbeat, are potential side effects. Even after intracardiac repair, there may occasionally be reduced blood flow to the lungs. If these difficulties persist, infants and children may need additional surgery, and in certain instances, artificial valves may be used to replace their natural pulmonary valves. Sometimes it takes decades after the initial operation to replace a pulmonary valve. As with any operation, there's also a chance of blood clots, unexpected bleeding, and infection. Although medicine is typically used to treat arrhythmias, some people may eventually require an implanted defibrillator or pacemaker. Throughout childhood, youth, and adulthood, complications may persist. Your child will require ongoing medical monitoring to detect and address any issues.

Continuous care

Your kid will need ongoing care following surgery. Your child will have regular check-ups scheduled by your doctor to ensure the treatment went well and to keep an eye out for any new issues.

Additionally, your child's doctor could advise limiting their physical activity. Your youngster might not be limited in their activities if the operation was a full success and there is no pulmonary valve leakage or obstruction.

CHAPTER THREE

Doctors may advise your child to take antibiotics before dental work in order to guard against infections that could lead to endocarditis, or inflammation of the heart's lining. However, in situations when the heart was fixed entirely, your child might not require prophylactic antibiotics. Nevertheless, people with prosthetic valves or those who have undergone repairs involving prosthetic materials are particularly advised to take preventive antibiotics. Consult a cardiologist about what is best for your child.

As your child gets older, you could be worried about the following aspects of child care:

avoiding infection. Preventive antibiotics may be necessary for a child with serious heart abnormalities prior to some dental and surgical treatments. To determine whether this is required, your doctor can assist you. Preventing infections can be effectively achieved by practicing proper oral hygiene and scheduling routine dental examinations.

Playing and exercising. Even after a successful course of treatment, parents of children with congenital heart abnormalities frequently worry about the hazards associated with rough play and vigorous activity. Many youngsters can lead regular or nearly normal lifestyles, even though others may need to restrict the type or quantity of exercise. Ask your child's doctor about safe activities for them to engage in; decisions on exercise should be made on an individual basis.

If you have congenital heart disease as an adult, you could be worried about things like:

Workplace. Generally speaking, a congenital cardiac abnormality won't restrict a person's employment prospects. It may not be advisable for an adult with severe heart rhythm issues or the possibility of life-threatening complications to pursue jobs that could endanger others, such bus or airplane driving.

maternity. Most congenital heart disease sufferers are able to carry out pregnancies without any issues. On the other hand, your chance of difficulties during pregnancy may increase if you have a serious defect or complications like arrhythmias or persistent pulmonary regurgitation.

Experts advise anyone with congenital heart disease who is thinking about having children to thoroughly evaluate the decision with their physician in advance. Consultations with medical professionals who specialize in cardiology, genetics, and high-risk obstetric care may be necessary prior to conception. Certain heart drugs may need to be stopped or changed before becoming pregnant because they are not safe to take while pregnant.

Adapting and providing assistance

Finding out that your child has potentially fatal cardiac abnormalities can be very terrifying. Talking to other parents, especially those who have previously had the operation, can offer you hope, encouragement, and someone to lean on, even though support groups aren't for everyone. Find out from your doctor whether your community has any parent support groups for kids with heart abnormalities.

Remember to occasionally give yourself a rest. Seek assistance from friends or relatives to help you look after your child. Try to arrange for friends and family to visit your child while they are in the hospital so you may return home for a shower, a nap, or some time with your other kids.

You might want to write down your child's diagnosis, prescriptions, dates of operations, and surgeries, as well as the name and phone number of your cardiologist, to help with care coordination. This note will help any new doctor understand your child's medical history and will give essential information to anyone else who could be caring for your child.

Make sure your new health insurance plan will pay for your child's care if you decide to switch, as some may not cover pre-existing conditions or may impose waiting periods.

THE END

www.ingramcontent.com/pod-product-compliance
Lightning Source LLC
Chambersburg PA
CBHW060823260726

48660CB00003B/1065